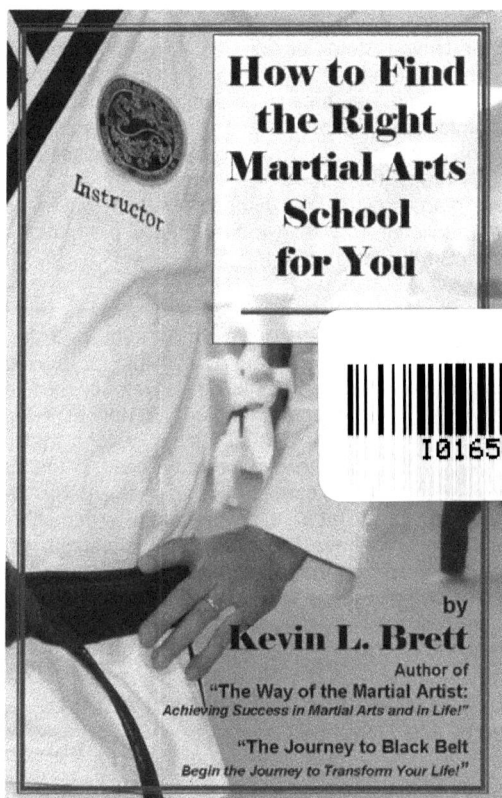

How to Find the Right Martial Arts School for You

Instructor

I0165020

by

Kevin L. Brett

Author of
"The Way of the Martial Artist:
Achieving Success in Martial Arts and in Life!"

"The Journey to Black Belt
Begin the Journey to Transform Your Life!"

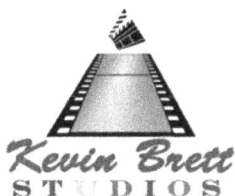

Kevin Brett
STUDIOS

Entertainment | Education | Family

www.KevinBrettStudios.com

How to Find the Right Martial Arts School for You

Publisher's Cataloging-In-Publication Data
(Prepared by The Donohue Group, Inc.)

Brett, Kevin L.
  How to Find the Right Martial Arts School for You/ Kevin L. Brett.

    p. : ill. ; cm.

    ISBN-13 9780981935058
    ISBN-10 0-9819350-5-2

1. Martial arts--Psychological aspects. 2. Martial arts. 3. Self-realization. 4. Mind and body. I. Title.

GV1102.7.P75 B74 2011
796.8   2011911902

ATTN: Quantity discounts are available to your company educational institution, government agency or martial arts organization.

For more information, please contact the author at Kevin Brett Studios, Inc.
19 Live Oak Lane, Stafford, Virginia 22554 540-845-4755
sales@KevinBrettStudios.com

Warning & Disclaimer

Marital arts can be lethal and the practice of martial arts or application of various martial arts techniques, training drills and exercises can cause serious injury or death. This book is intended for informational and entertainment purposes. It is not intended as a substitute for a specific martial arts training program by a qualified martial arts school or instructor. You should consult a qualified physician before engaging in any exercise program or physical activities to ascertain whether you or the other participants are mentally and physically healthy enough to engage in such activities.

Martial arts are for defensive purposes only and should be used only as a last resort and only with the least amount of force or technique necessary to reduce the immediate threat or risk in a self-defense situation. Anyone applying fighting or martial arts techniques or methods could be liable in civil or criminal court. You must control your actions and remain within the boundaries of the laws of the jurisdiction in which any defensive techniques may be employed.

The author, publisher and sellers of this book assume no liability for personal injury or damage to property as a result of practicing any concepts or content represented or implied within this book. All individuals are responsible for their own actions. The author, publisher and sellers of this book also provide no warranty or guarantee, expressed or implied that the techniques, concepts or content presented in this book will be effective in any or all self-defense situations.

Do You Have Everything You Need to Succeed in the Martial Arts and in Life?

Kevin Brett Studios is the author of, the book, *"The Way of the Martial Artist: Achieving Success in Martial Arts and in Life!"*

(240 pp., $11.95, ISBN-13: 978-0981935003), available from Amazon.com, BarnesandNobel.com, Books.Google.com for Kindle or from the author's website www.KevinBrettStudios.com and other retailers. This book helps readers what is likely lacking in their training, and what it means to have a well-rounded martial arts

education. Certified Martial Arts Instructor Kevin Brett provides insights into the origins, skills, training methods, strategies, tactics and character and spirit of the martial artist. This book is jammed with motivation, inspiration and education for martial artists from beginners to master-level and it culminates with the chapter: Success for Life which provides readers with seventeen techniques to incorporate in your training and your every day life to achieve your most important goals. It also covers the five elements of success and teaches you how to develop your own personal blueprint for translating the achievements, discipline and success factors you achieve in martial arts into every other aspect of your life!

Martial arts are about survival and this book teaches readers how to develop the skill, strategy and character of a true martial artist to supplement their dojo training. It also provides in-depth insight into just what students and parents want from martial arts: discipline, commitment, honor, respect, perseverance and ultimately – success in any life-undertaking. Kevin Brett provides answers and insights to questions that all martial artists ask during their quest for excellence, purpose and enlightenment.

The Way of the Martial Artist: Achieving Success in Martial Arts and in Life! uses the principles of martial arts to show readers how any worthwhile goal or life challenge can be approached and achieved with black belt determination. The servant-warrior is an ancient concept that the author re-introduces to help modern readers understand how any success should be a service or benefit to others.

Shawn Kovacich, author of the highly acclaimed book series ***Achieving Kicking Excellence*** and high-ranking martial artist, calls ***The Way of the Martial Artist***, *"A comprehensive framework of the numerous principles and concepts you will need to become the best martial artist that* *you can be."* Black belt Richard Hefner says, *"The Way of the Martial Artist is part success manual, part martial arts guide and part survival guide, and all essential!"*

Lawrence Kane, author of **Surviving Armed Assaults** and **Martial Arts Instruction**; co-author of **The Way of Kata**, **The Way to Black Belt**, and The **Little Black Book of Violence** says, *"Kevin Brett has written an informative, interesting and useful book that I wholeheartedly recommend."*

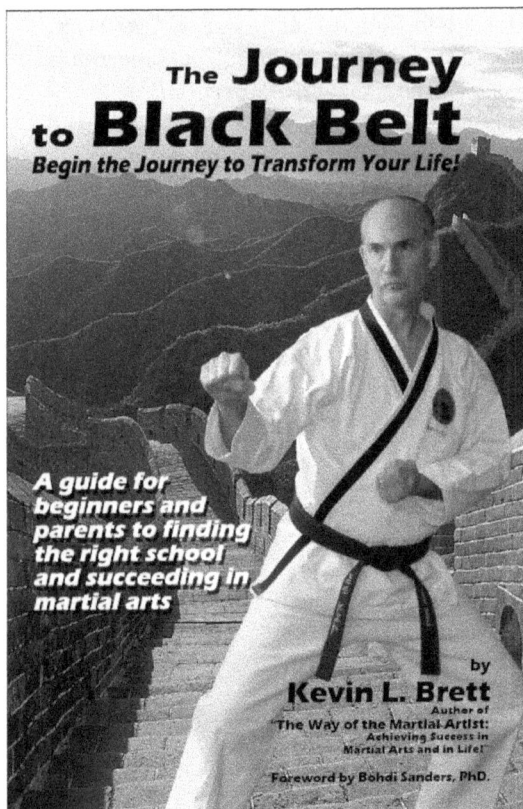

The **Journey** to **Black Belt**

Begin the Journey to Transform Your Life!

A guide for beginners and parents to finding the right school and succeeding in martial arts

by
Kevin L. Brett
Author of
*The Way of the Martial Artist:
Achieving Success in
Martial Arts and in Life!*

Foreword by Bohdi Sanders, PhD.

(223 pp., $11.95, ISBN-13: 978-0981935041), available from Amazon.com, BarnesandNobel.com, Books.Google.com for Kindle or from the author's website www.KevinBrettStudios.com and other retailers.

Kevin Brett's book is the perfect book for anyone who is interested in getting into the martial arts or getting their children started in the martial arts. *The Journey to Black Belt* covers everything that a potential student needs to know in order to make an informed decision when it comes to selecting the right martial arts style, school, and instructor. He explains the difference in the individual martial arts, as well as guides the reader concerning what he or she should look for when trying to decide on the right instructor. Mr. Brett even covers things such as discovering your true goals and how to achieve your goals.

The book is organized much like an outline with short topic sections throughout. I personally find books which are formatted in this style, especially guide books or resource books, much easier to read and follow. The format and style of this book is perfect. This is, without a doubt, the most complete book of its kind on the market. I really can't think of anything that a potential martial arts student would need to know that *The Journey to Black Belt* leaves out. It is simply that complete!

Bohdi Sanders, Ph.D.
Author:
Wisdom of the Elders,
Wicked Wisdom: Explorations into the Dark Side,
Life Lessons: Politically Incorrect Wisdom,
Fireside Meditations
www.TheWisdomWarrior.com

How to Find the Right Martial Arts School for You

Contents

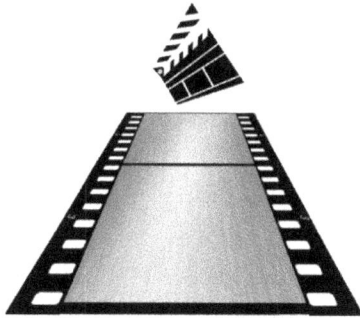

Kevin Brett
STUDIOS

Entertainment | Education | Family

www.KevinBrettStudios.com

How to Find the Right Martial Arts School for You

Introduction

"Warriors are expected to be servants of society and people of virtue."

My name is Kevin Brett. I am a certified Martial Arts Instructor with more than twenty years of training and teaching experience in the martial arts and the author of *"The Way of the Martial Artist: Achieving Success in Martial Arts and in Life!"* and *"The Journey to Black Belt"*.

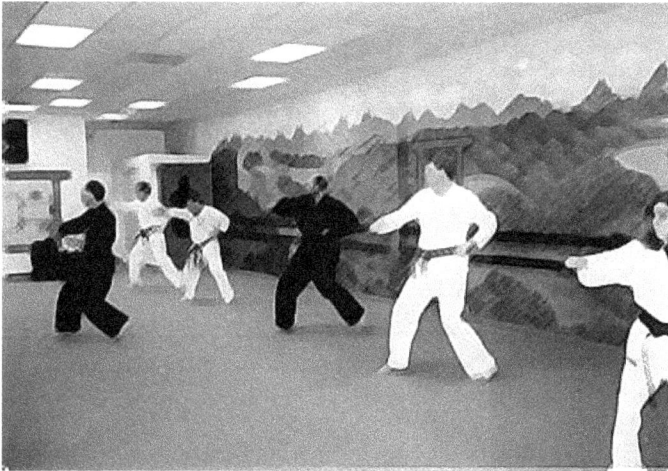

I have developed this new book *"How to Find the Right Martial Arts School for You"* to help beginning martial artists and you parents who are considering involving your children in the world of martial arts. My hope is that the ideas and information I share in these pages will help you to become more knowledgeable about martial arts schools, how to find a good school.

To the outsider, trying to understand and get started in martial arts can be confusing, mysterious and even frustrating. The information in this book will help you or your child get off to a great start in the exciting world of martial arts. Shopping for a school involves understanding the benefits, how to know when you've found a good school and a style and how to sort your way through all the marketing and advertising hype.

Martial arts can be one of the most rewarding undertakings of your life. The confidence and character that result from achieving such an objective are difficult to match in any other endeavor. Martial arts are indeed a lifelong journey that can continue to provide endless rewards. Like life, martial arts present challenges and opportunities for growth. How we handle these challenges is key. If we handle them well, we will grow in character, stature and maturity and reach new levels of personal excellence. If we handle them poorly and do not learn the lessons that are there for us to experience, we risk stumbling down a path that can lead to frustration, disappointment and failure.

There are many benefits to be gained from martial arts study for both children and adults. Parents typically expect martial arts schools to instill key virtues such as respect, discipline, goal-setting, determination and of-course, self-defense and fitness. There are many styles of martial arts; many masters, many schools and many training methods from which to choose. There are also many different types of martial arts programs and memberships and payment plans. A little education in the whole matter will go a long way to helping you feel more confident in whatever decision you make.

I have designed this book to help the beginner understand three main things:

- **How to Get Started:** *understanding what martial arts is about and the differences between strictly learning self-defense, vs. some recognized style of martial arts*
- **Self-Defense vs. Traditional Martial Arts**
- **Martial Styles:** *the differences between the various styles*
- **Shopping for a School and Style of Martial Art:** *How to shop with confidence for a martial arts school and know what you're getting*

I would also recommend you consider obtaining a copy of my book *"The Way of the Martial Artist: Achieving Success in Martial Arts and in Life!"* and *"The Journey to Black Belt: Begin the Journey to*

Transform Your Life!" to accompany you as you begin your journey in the martial arts. Many notable martial artists have highly recommended these books as invaluable guides for martial artists.

I hope the end result of reading this book about finding the right school is that you feel much more educated and confident about searching for a school so that you know what to expect. I hope the process of selecting a given style to study.

☯ Chapter 1

Getting Started in Martial Arts

"If you want to change your life, then you need to trade in your wishbone for a backbone and get started!"

Tips for Parents

Lot's of parents have found karate offers their children many benefits they cannot find in other athletic activities. Martial arts do not happen overnight. Your child will not become a virtuoso pianist overnight, nor will they become a stellar black belt after a few weeks of lessons, but they will progress over time if they are committed. The first thing parents need to understand is that most people -- especially children -- are not able to train every day. Martial arts are like studying. The best results come from working at a steady pace -- not from cramming. Sports psychologists call this distributed practice versus massed practice. I call it common sense.

Most children will quickly tire of something if they do it every day. Martial arts are no exception. Parents help your children by fostering a training schedule that results in two or three lessons or classes every week. This kind of schedule prevents burnout. It gives the body a chance to rebuild properly. So, I encourage you to set a regular schedule that allows your child to progress steadily instead of cramming at the last minute. Hopefully this same concept will carry over into their school and studies as well. A good habit can be applied in multiple areas of life!

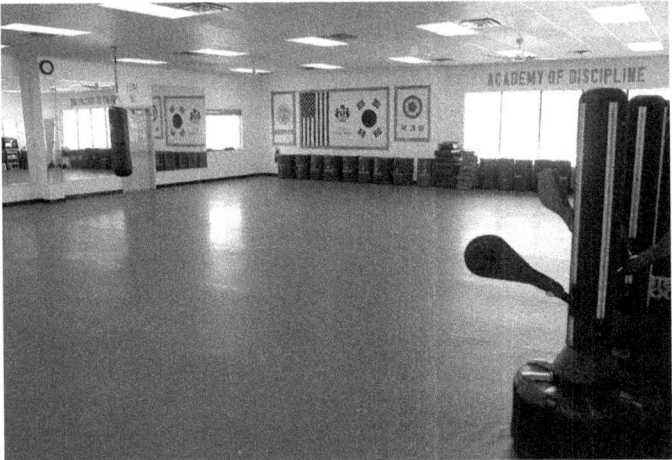

A typical Tae Kwon Do Dojang; flags, mirrors, pads, kicks pads along the far wall – the basics

It's also important to get your child to class on time. This means wearing the uniform, or allowing a few extra minutes to change. Again, this will help them develop good habits of planning ahead and more effectively managing their time.

There are some other important tips that will help your child progress; one includes his or her uniform. Both the belt and the uniform deserve respect. In martial arts, the belt is a symbol of accomplishment, as well as rank. The uniform is a symbol of training and hard work. Children should not play in their uniforms and should treat their belt with respect. When they are in the Dojang, Dojo, or training hall, they must follow the rules of the school. This includes neat and clean dress.

Positive reinforcement is very important. When your child does something well, make a point of mentioning it. Always praise your child for his or her efforts. Praise encourages good performance and helps build the child's sense of self-esteem which is an essential ingredient to a happy and successful life.

Just as parent involvement is important in an academic setting, your interest and cooperation will speed your child's progress in martial arts. Again, it is important to remember that most things in life -- including martial arts -- require time and hard work to achieve mastery. There are no overnight wonders in the martial arts world.

Hard work, patience, praise, communication and cooperation will result in progress for your child. By helping our children reach their potential, we are improving the quality of life not just for them, but for everyone. Remember... they are the future!

Martial Arts Today

Martial arts in the 21st century are concerned more with the practical application of techniques, sport and competition. However, martial arts study for adults and children has retained many of the core values of martial arts of old. The values associated with martial arts study are like the interwoven threads that hold society together. The values include respect, perseverance, self-discipline, self-respect, kindness, tolerance, honesty and loyalty.

Much of the deterioration, crime and moral decay in today's society can be directly linked to a deterioration in core values. Where there is an absence of these values there are serious problems. Martial arts study and the pursuit of martial arts goals entails development and enhancement of these core values within the student. This system has been proven countless times to benefit children in their formative years and adults as well.

Martial arts students, whether child or adult, quickly learn the value of hard work, determination, honesty, and respect. They also learn many other qualities that are necessary for being happy with themselves and successful in their lives; that is a key theme in my book, **"The Way of the Martial Artist: Achieving Success in**

Martial Arts and in Life!" In short, to study martial arts is to learn to be the master of oneself.

As a student, you will develop true self-confidence from accomplishing your goals in martial arts. You will learn the value of setting goals and maintaining consistent effort to accomplish them. That is a quality that will serve you or your child for a lifetime.

The confidence and character that many students develop is amazing and the transformation is for life. Often, they find that they are not easily tempted or influenced by peer pressure. Students learn to avoid rather than resort to violent solutions to problems and conflicts in their lives. With their newfound self-confidence many students are motivated to take on new challenges in their life. For some it may be beginning a new sport that they had never considered themselves able to handle. For others it may be taking on new challenges and roles of leadership and responsibility in their work, school or other career activities.

Martial arts is much more than simply kicking and punching; it is the development of the character and the improvement of self. Students improve their work or study habits and many students reach heights that they had never thought possible. Perseverance allows a student to continue to pass through levels of self-realization that would have never been possible otherwise. As I mentioned in *"The Way of the Martial Artist"* – *"To achieve your dreams, you must leave your comfort zone and never return."*

Commitment

Black belts are just ordinary people, but with extraordinary commitment and that's what sets them apart. You will never achieve success in anything until you are committed to it. I can't tell you how many people walked through our doors at United Karate and expressed great interest in martial arts. They would not think twice about spending a lot of time describing their fascination and admiration of martial arts and those who study them. That is where their involvement in martial arts ended. They stopped in essentially to tell us that they were interested admirers.

Other visitors simply walked in and said, "Where do I sign?" So what's the difference? Simple, one was interested and the other was committed. Now do you see? Our society is full of dreamers and doers, and a rare, lucky few are blessed to have both qualities. Dreaming and doing ultimately lead to success; whether it's earning your black belt, climbing the corporate ladder or achieving some other meaningful and challenging personal goal. Commitment keeps you going when you begin to waiver. There will be slumps and setbacks, you will reach plateaus and maybe even a few brick walls, but persistence will eventually get you there. Commit to your own success and keep that commitment fresh and clear in your mind and you will travel far!

☯ Chapter 2

Self-Defense vs. Martial Arts

"If you can't defense yourself ... nothing else matters."

The Practical Need for Self-Defense

Effective and lethal self-defense training need not take the many years it can take to earn a black belt and in fact, in most instances will be more effective than typical commercial black belt training which puts much emphasis on sport competition and simply learning the forms, patterns or kata as set routine with little if any practical and proven self-defense application of the techniques being taught.

Many of the techniques taught in self-defense classes can cause serious injury or even death to an assailant, so it is crucial to have only serious, mature students. This training is ideal for a wide range of individuals who would readily benefit from acquiring basic self-defense skills. These skills will help students develop confidence and competence in threatening situations.

Violence in our schools is increasing at an alarming rate. High school and college students simply must be capable of defending themselves. Young mothers, young men, and even middle-aged and older individuals are all potential beneficiaries of this type of training because no one is immune to threatening situations.

Truly effective self defense techniques require minimal strength and capitalize on the application of leverage and knowledge of vital areas. This makes these techniques ideal for many individuals, especially women who typically have less upper body strength than men.

The most effective self defense techniques are simple to execute and easy to learn. In a real self defense situation there is no time for complex techniques or motion picture style theatrics. The objective is simply to use the least force needed to allow the student to free themselves from the threat and escape from the scene of an assault.

Modern Self-Defense Training

I hope for your own safety that you are not one of those incredibly naïve folks who think you are big enough and strong enough to defend yourself and that's all you need or that you don't hang out in bad, dangerous areas, so you don't have anything to worry about. Those are exactly the types of people who need self-defense training the most. They are living under some seriously flawed assumptions and they don't even suspect that they are at risk. That very attitude puts them more at risk because they refuse to believe they are in any danger. Nothing could be further from the truth. Quit burying your head in the sand like an Ostrich and look around you. A violent assault is committed somewhere in the United States every seven seconds. That's a lot of victims, or as I prefer to view it, a lot of potential survivors.

You do not have to be a black belt to be able to defend yourself. Many people have the misconception that in order to adequately defend themselves they must be built like Arnold Schwartzeneger or that they must be some world class black belt capable of breaking a dozen bricks with their forehead. Nothing could be further from the truth. Below are a few basic tenets of self-defense that are vital to your survival.

What is Self-Defense?

1. Self-defense is any technique, tactic or strategy that can be used to neutralize an assailant and escape.
2. Self-defense can employ defensive use of anything from hand-to-hand combat, clawing, scratching, biting, spitting, using pepper spray, knives, everyday objects used as makeshift weapons of opportunity, the victim's immediate environment or firearms.
3. The most effective self-defense techniques require minimal strength and take advantage of leverage and knowledge of vital targets on the body.
4. Effective self-defense techniques are simple and easy to learn and can include kicking, stomping, choking, grappling, gouging, poking, biting and any other method that gets the job done.

A basic self-defense program should include awareness training where students are taught specific methods for avoiding and recognizing potentially dangerous situations or individuals before trouble starts. As in medicine, prevention is the best medicine. If a student can avoid a possible assault or confrontation, that is the best self defense of all. You want to learn the psychology of defending yourself even before trouble actually starts.

For those situations where alertness or psychology are not sufficient to deal with the problem, basic self-defense training should include escape maneuvers for the most common types of grabs, chokes and holds, more advanced defensive moves to combat punches and kicks, and counters for armed attacks.

In a purely self-defense program you will not be taught to become a martial artist in the traditional sense with belts and ranks. You are simply learning a vocabulary of self defense techniques with which you can respond to situations that you are likely to encounter.

In addition to escape techniques, you should learn techniques and drills for striking and disabling an assailant. In the domain of self defense, techniques typically fall into one of two categories: destructive, disabling techniques and non-destructive controlling techniques. Destructive techniques are intended to maim or kill. They are only used as a desperate last resort after first attempting to diffuse the situation with non-destructive, controlling techniques which allow the victim to escape, but ultimately leave the assailant free of permanent injuries.

Continue and learn more advanced self-defense techniques and then consider training in a traditional martial art. Continuation in a traditional martial arts belt system will significantly enhance your physical conditioning, skill levels, confidence and knowledge, however, there are a number of self-defense options in most metropolitan areas.

Red Man type classes are popular. Essentially, these classes involve a human target, the aggressor, dressed in martial arts protective padded gear from head to toe. Class members learn basic strikes, punches, kicks and the like and are able to practice against a live aggressor who attempts to attack them. The quality of these classes varies greatly, but check and see what is available in your area. If you are serious about learning some very basic concepts and techniques quickly to kick start your skills, this may be an option prior to more structure learning in something like a traditional martial arts school.

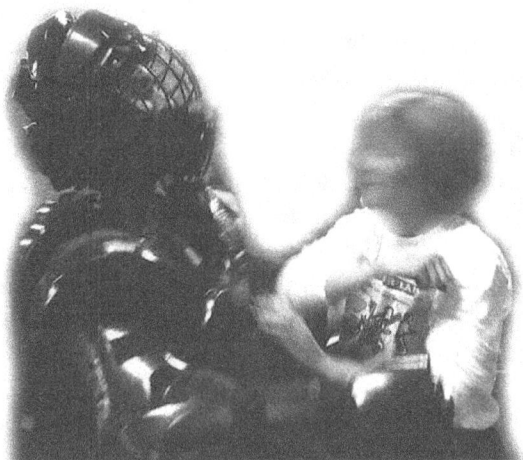

Krav Maga – the Israeli system of self-defense is not a traditional martial art. While some Krav Maga schools do incorporate a belt system, this is not how the system was originally structured. Nonetheless, there are a number of variants of Krav Maga including Commando Krav Maga and so forth. There are a growing number of Krav Maga organizations that have splintered off from the original system and some of them offer instructor certification programs. Check your local area for options or even consult your local police or sheriff department to see what they recommend.

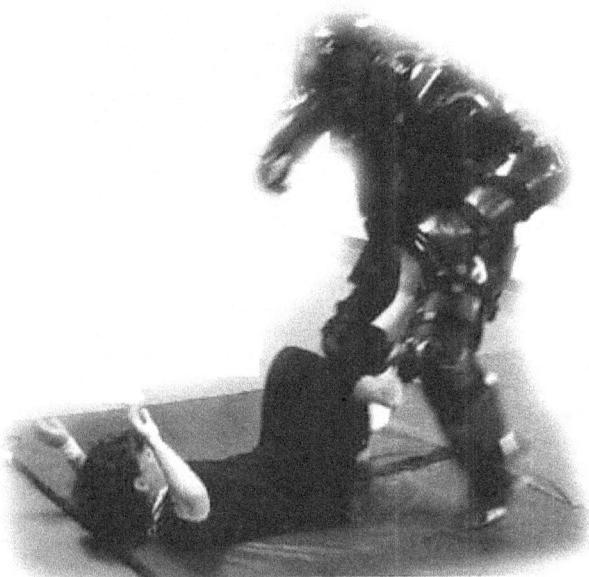

A self-defense class where participants strike a heavily padded assailant in realistic assault situations

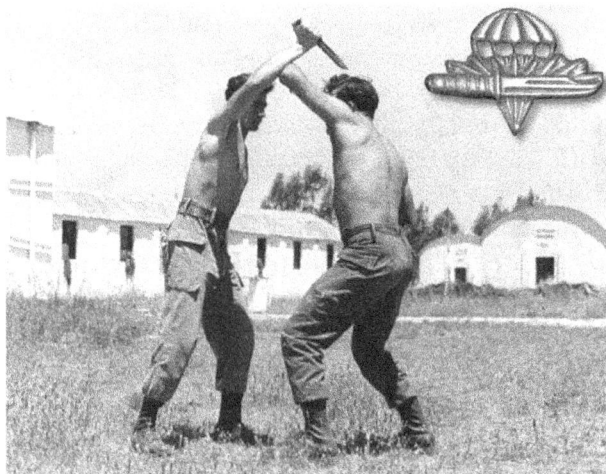

Israeli Commandos practice Krav Maga

Realism

The more realistic the training experience ...the less shocking reality will seem. Part of varying your training is practicing for realism. Take your training seriously. If it is a joke or becomes too much of a social gathering, you will be easily surprised or overwhelmed in a real situation. Some schools

19

of martial arts practice in swamps, rain, and all types of terrain and environments. Martial arts are a war fighting skill where realism is a key ingredient in training. Part of the reason for the diversity and variation in training is to introduce different realistic elements. A curious thing happens when you make a training drill very realistic, you become uncomfortable. In the Marine Corps Martial Arts Program (MCMAP) and in many traditional martial arts schools across the world, some aspects of the training are conducted in realistic settings, rain, snow, and sand, in shallow streams or ponds and in uneven terrain. Some training is at night and all of these conditions are intended to simulate reality and the conditions in which a student, soldier or law enforcement officer might find themselves having to apply their martial arts skills.

At United Karate we used to take students out into the parking light occasionally and have them dressed in street clothes. We would have other senior in students hiding behind cars and positioned in other hiding spots ready to leap out and simulate an assault on the students in training so that they could get used to working in confined spaces such as between cars or at night with limited lighting and visibility. The point was to make the training a challenge and then see how the students performed. Every one appreciated the dose of reality. Reality isn't always pleasant, but reality is what you are training for. Being uncomfortable is a good thing. Get used to it in training so that you will not be surprised if it happens for real.

Child Safety

Self-defense for children is a challenging subject. There are books and videos available that teach techniques, but the reality is that an adult male or female of even average strength can physically overcome a young child. At United Karate we began teaching self-defense techniques to students beginning at age twelve because this is typically the midst of the middle-school years where children are often the meanest to each other. In elementary school, what few physical altercations might occur can be dealt with by using the basic kicks, punches or blocks taught by most martial arts styles. Of course this is only a last resort when the child feels physically threatened by another child of approximately the same age.

To address the issue of responding to a much larger, stronger child or adult assailant, I prefer to focus on one very simple acronym as a memory and training aid. **Fire and G.E.T. Out**. (Groin, Eyes, Throat). It's an incredibly simple approach. First, other adults generally will not turn their head to notice if another child is screaming for help or yelling "stop!" We're simply exposed to too many instances of children playing around or joking or simply becoming angry with each other to respond every time we hear this plea for help. When someone yells "Fire" however, we don't hear that everyday and our subconscious is programmed from a very early age to fear fire and its effects. That typically makes a much more effective plea for help.

The G.E.T portion tells your child what they must do; strike the assailants, groin, eyes and throat in any order with any weapon, punch, chop or poke they can. Strike one or all of these targets many times, strike hard and strike fast. Even the strongest adult can be distracted, injured or disabled if your child focuses on those three targets. Your child's hands or arms may be pinned or held, but at some point during the assault they can hopeful have a second where they may be free to strike – that is the chance they must watch for. It might just save their life!

It is also important for children to be taught concepts of street awareness and playground safety as well as school safety and what to do in tragic situations such as school shootings.

☯ Chapter 3

Martial Arts Styles

"On any given day a well-trained martial artist of one style can defeat a well-trained martial artist of another style. There really is no single 'best' style. It depends upon you!"

Studying marital arts without having some familiarity with the origins of your own style or the history of martial arts in general is like being a member of your family and knowing nothing of your heritage or family history. A well-rounded martial artist should have some appreciation of the roots of the thing he is spending so much effort studying.

Understanding Martial Arts Styles

There are literally hundreds of martial arts styles originating in countries like Korea, Japan, China, Burma, the Philippines, Okinawa, Brazil and others. At the core of all of the many styles from each of these countries is an approach toward self-defense. The differences are typically in the general types of techniques that are emphasized in a given style. The founder or creator of a given style developed his style based on some philosophy of defense. Different styles were developed with different influences from their creators.

Some styles are based on animal or insect movements that gave clues to their creators about different styles of movement and defensive tactics. Other styles are based on a philosophy of attack and defense that is built upon by an assortment of techniques intended to defend against certain types of attacks against various types of weapons. The next section describes how some of these styles have evolved into martial arts organizations and what some of the philosophical differences are between styles.

The important thing to take away from this is that there is no one style that is better than another. It all depends upon the self-defense situation, the skill level of the defender and the choice of techniques used in a defensive situation. Do not be fooled by school owners or masters who get involved in heated debates about who's style is best. They are all art forms. Go to an art gallery and decide which painting is the best. It is all a matter of opinion and perspective. I would simply encourage you to study a little bit about several common styles and learn about their general types of techniques and training methods. Different styles are sometimes better suited to different physical builds of people, but this is not always the case. Hit the internet and learn a little before you commit to a style or school.

You'll feel more comfortable about your decision once you do choose a school.

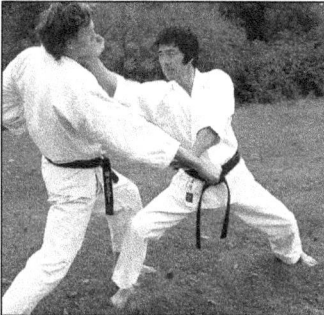

Martial Style: Karate-do and Shotokan
Country: Japan
Characteristics: Hard strikes, kicks, block, grappling similar to Tae Kwon Do

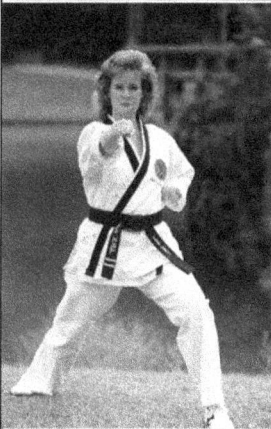

Martial Style: Tae Kwon Do
Country: Korea
Characteristics: Punches, many different types of kicks, hand strikes and blocks, grappling, practical schools teach destructive combat application or bunkai of the movements in hyungs (forms or poomse)

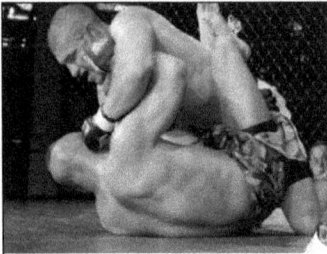

Martial Style: Mixed Martial Arts
Country: USA
Characteristics: Grappling, sweeps, throws, punches, kicks, ground fighting

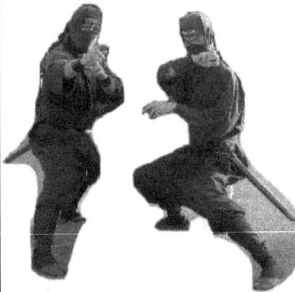

Martial Style: Ninjutsu (Ninja style)
Country: Japan
Characteristics: Typically involves basic strikes, punches hand techniques, throws, take-downs, special weapons and tactics

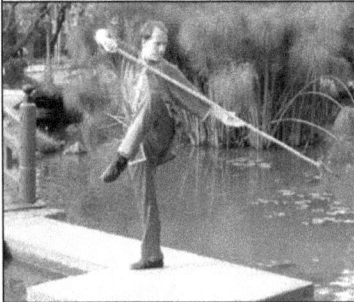

Martial Style: Wushu
Country: China
Characteristics: Many weapons and rapid circular blocks and strike combinations mixed with straight blocks and strikes

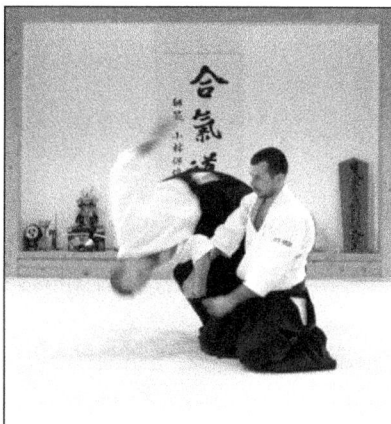

Martial Style: Aikido
Country: Japan
Characteristics: Typically non-destructive techniques involving grappling, sweeps and other take-downs and throws, joint locks and joint manipulation, often using your opponent's force against them.

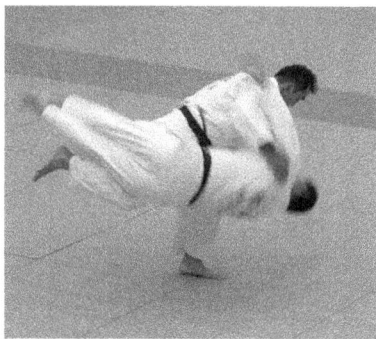

Martial Style: Judo
Country: Japan
Characteristics: Grappling, throws, sweeps and other takedowns, ground fighting, joint locks, typically non-destructive techniques

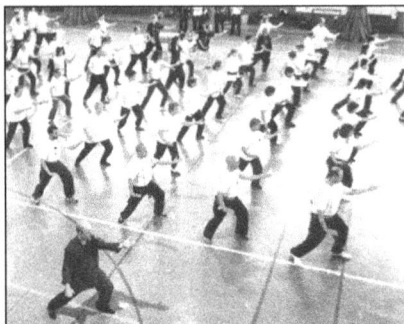

Martial Style: Tai Chi
Country: China
Characteristics: Smooth flowing techniques typically practiced in slow motion, but with combat application. Some styles use the Tai Chi sword and other weapons.

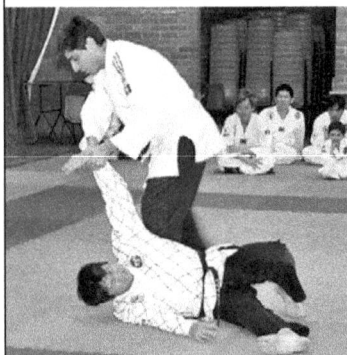

Martial Style: Hapkido
Country: Korea
Characteristics: Grappling, throws, sweeps and other take-downs sword, kicks, joint locks and manipulation

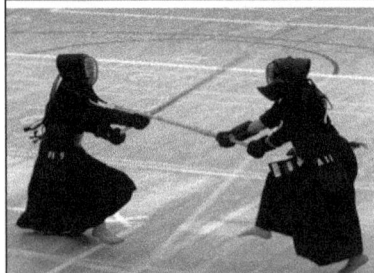

Martial Style: Kendo
Country: Japan
Characteristics: Uses the shinai, bamboo practice sword, effectively sport swordsmanship based on Samurai tradition

Fighting Systems and Martial Arts

Martial arts have a spiritual and ethical foundation and a governing philosophy, fighting systems do not. For example, Krav Maga (a Hebrew term meaning close combat) is the Israeli system of self-defense used by the Israeli military. It is very effective and deadly like many martial arts, but it is a fighting system rather than a martial art. It consists of tactical concepts and techniques, some overall guiding principles for engaging in combat and nothing more. It is highly effective, but it has no philosophical component or spiritual aspect to it.

A martial art may contain philosophical elements that train an artist to avoid confrontation or mitigate risk. It will prepare you to consider carefully the fact that you are about to cause serious or even fatal consequences to an aggressor who is still another human being. By contrast, a fighting system will simply address the fact that an aggressive act has occurred which requires an appropriate physical response. There is no consideration other than to cause maximum damage to the other individual. More of the key elements of character, spirit and philosophy will be covered later.

Every martial art has a ranking system as do some self-defense systems or fighting systems. Many of the Japanese systems are similar to each other. Some of the Korean systems such as Tae Kwon Do are similar to Japanese. The Chinese systems have their own different means of rank and identification.

Every martial artist should at least have some familiarity with other systems.

The Legend of the Belts

In ancient times martial arts students began their studies with a white uniform and a white belt. The belt was used not only as a symbol of rank, but to hold up their pants as well. Many martial arts classes were held outdoors or in a Dojang that may have had only a dirt floor. As students continued in their studies, their white belts would begin to turn yellow with the sweat from their workouts. As they worked outdoors in the grass, rolling, flipping and practicing take downs, their belts would take on green stains. As the students worked during the course of several years their 'white' belts became more soiled with blood, dirt and mud. Eventually, when the student tested before the headmaster of the school they would be presented with a black belt if they passed. At that point students were allowed to also wear black uniforms if they choose.

As students progressed from beginning levels to expert level, their belts became darker. After reaching the black belt level a student was then beginning all over again on a higher level. Black belts would train, study and teach to reach higher levels of knowledge, proficiency and martial skill. As the new black belt began to wear with age, it would fray and show the white material inside of the belt reminding even the most experienced black belts that they are all still white belt students inside.

Today we use a colored belt system to signify the level of skill of progress of the student. The belt colors get progressively darker as the student works towards the black belt level. The black stripes on the belt are used to mark a student's progress in their requirements for their belt level.

Earning a new belt in the martial arts is a significant achievement for anyone. Students should always remember that unlike many other things in life, a new belt in Karate is not automatic or guaranteed; it must be earned, the old fashioned way, with hard work and determination: Nothing really worth doing is ever easy, but the rewards are certainly worth the effort required.

Always treat your belt and other student's belts with respect. Tradition has it that a student should never wash their belt because that would be like washing out the sweat and work that went into earning it! Of course you should always wash and press your uniform as a sign of respect to your instructors. Your uniform should be treated with respect because it is a training tool and a part of your martial arts equipment. All of your martial arts equipment, manuals, videos, bags, uniforms, sparring gear and weapons should be kept in neat clean condition. Keeping your equipment in ready condition helps students develop the necessary discipline required to always be prepared.

Typical Meanings for the Different Belt Colors

In most martial arts systems that incorporate colored belt ranks, there are various meaning associated with the particular colors of the different belts. The table below includes common meanings of the belts in the Tae Kwon Do family of styles. There are many variations, but this should give you some idea of the concept of progression of knowledge, skill and maturity.

Belt Color	Meaning
White	The student is pure or without knowledge of Tae Kwon Do.
Yellow	Symbolizes the student, likened to a seed, is beginning to see the sunlight.
Orange	Represents the full power of the sun, or knowledge which will help the seed take root.
Light Green	Represents the seed beginning to grow.
Dark Green	Shows the young seedling flourishing.
Blue	Designates the young plant reaching for the sky.
Purple	Represents the clouds of rain which feed the plant and give it life.
Red	Signifies Danger. The student has good technical knowledge, but still lacks control and discipline.
Brown	Symbolizes closeness to earth, or a better

	understanding of one's mind and body.
Black	Means no fear of the dark, or an understanding of the art. There are 9 degrees of Black Belt. When all the above colors are combined in equal amounts, they come out black. Black represents the combination of all of the knowledge gained from all of the belts which come before.

Since Take Kwon Do is the most widespread style in the United States and for the most part, around the world, I have provided a brief history of this art.

Brief History of Tae Kwon Do

The kwans or schools of Tae Kwon Do were born after World War II as the masters of these new styles established their schools. Jhoon Rhee was the first to accurately document (1969 Action Karate) the development of the Kwans in Korea. Master Rhee is the father of American Tae Kwon Do.

According to Jhoon Rhee the first five Kwans were: Chung Do Kwan(1945), Moo Duk Kwan, which taught Tang Soo Do (1945), Yun Moo Kwan (1945), Chang Moo Kwan (1946), Chi Do Kwan (1946). Several more Kwans were founded after 1953 and in the early 1960s. The chart below show the major Kwans of Tae Kwon Do:

```
                        ┌─────────────────┐
                        │    TAEKYON      │
                        └────────┬────────┘
        ┌────────────┬──────────┼──────────┬────────────┐
┌──────────────┐ ┌──────────────┐ ┌──────────────┐ ┌──────────────┐
│ Chung do kwan│ │ Moo duk kwan │ │ Yun moo kwan │ │  Chi do kwan │
│    1945      │ │    1945      │ │    1945      │ │    1946      │
└──────────────┘ └──────────────┘ └──────────────┘ └──────────────┘
    ┌──────────────┬──────────────┐     ┌──────────────┬──────────────┐
┌──────────────┐ ┌──────────────┐ ┌──────────────┐ ┌──────────────┐
│Song moo kwan/│ │ Ji do kwan/  │ │Chang moo kwan│ │  Oh do kwan  │
│Sang moo kwan │ │ Jee do kwan  │ │    1946      │ │   1953-54    │
│   1953-54    │ │   1953-54    │ └──────────────┘ └──────────────┘
└──────────────┘ └──────────────┘
                        ┌─────────────────────────┐
                        │      TAE KWON DO         │
                        │ (Formed April 11, 1955)  │
                        └─────────────────────────┘
```

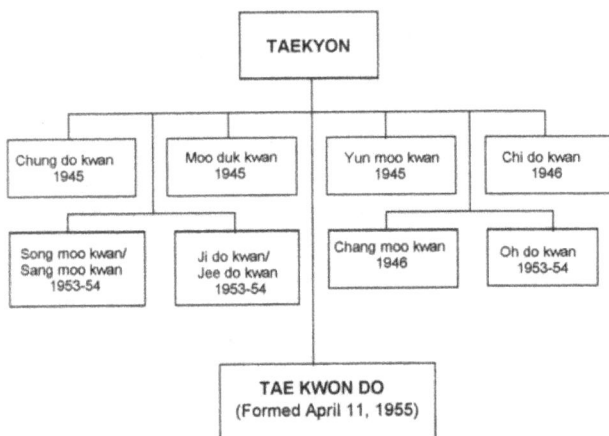

The eight original Kwans of Tae Kwon Do

In 1945 the new Korean military was established. Choi Hong Hi, then a second lieutenant in the army, began teaching Taekyon to Korean army troops. Later Choi gave Taekyon demonstrations during training in Kansas which was the first exhibition of this style in the United States.

A movement developed from 1945 to 1955 to unite the martial arts of Korea into one system. Finally, in 1955, a conference of Chung Do Kwan masters adopted the term Tae Kwon Do coined by Choi Hong Hi, who had risen to the rank of general. The name was chosen by General Choi because of its similarity to Taekyon.

In 1952 a demonstration was given to Korean President Syngman Rhee. As a result of this demonstration

34

Syngman Rhee decreed that all Korean soldiers be trained in the martial arts. In 1954 General Choi Hong Hi developed a center for Taekyon training for the Korean military on the island of Che Ju.

In 1961, by order of the new military government, the Korean Tae Kwon Do association (KTA) was established with General Choi Hong Hi as its first President. The KTA established national standards for black belt certification.

General Choi sent Tae Kwon Do practitioners to many countries to internationalize the art. Jhoon Rhee was the first to introduce Tae Kwon Do in the United States in 1956 at San Marcos Southwest Texas State College. He was attending college where he taught a non-accredited Tae Kwon Do course. In 1958 he founded his first public Tae Kwon Do club in San Marcos.

Tae Kwon Do proliferated in Korea from the military to the public school system. Many public Dojangs were established and Tae Kwon Do was accepted as a required part of physical education training in the public schools.

General Choi Hong Hi founded the International Tae Kwon Do Federation in 1966, resigned from the KTA and moved to Saskatchuan, Canada.

The South Vietnamese government asked for help from General Hi to provide instructors to teach their troops Tae Kwon Do to help in their struggle with the North

Vietnamese. Tae Kwon Do spread to other parts of the Pacific rim, Europe, the Netherlands and the Middle East.

In 1968 Tae Kwon Do made its way to Britain, Spain, Belgium, India, Yugoslavia and Hungary. In 1973 the World Tae Kwon Do Federation (WTF) was established back in Tae Kwon Do's home country of Korea. In 1974 the U.S. Tae Kwon Do Federation was formed.

Jhoon Rhee invented the original safety chops for competition sparring and eventually opened the first Tae Kwon Do school in the former Soviet Union after the fall of Communism. He was also a major influence in the movement to make Tae Kwon Do an Olympic sport.

Under the direction of General Hi, Tae Kwon Do has spread to more than 62 countries. It is estimated there are 15 million Tae Kwon Do practitioners, far exceeding any other single art. In 1975 more than 700,000 were reported to be practicing in the U.S alone. Today there are many millions Tae Kwon Do students in the United States!

In 1980 the International Olympic Committee (IOC) recognized Tae Kwon Do as a legitimate Olympic sport. As a result Tae Kwon Do was a part of the Olympic Games in Seoul Korea in 1988 with the United States Olympic Tae Kwon Do Team taking the gold medal!

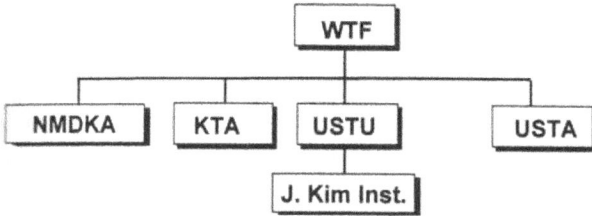

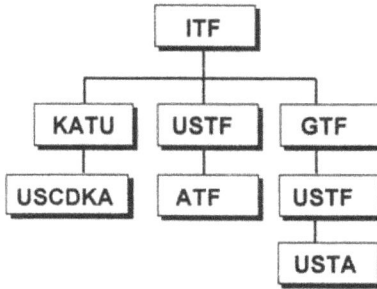

Tae Kwon Do Organizations

Internationally Recognized:

- ITF - International TKD Federation (Chonji forms)
- KATU - KoreAmerican TKD Union (Chonji forms)
- GTF - Global TDK Federation (Chonji forms)
- USTF - United States TKD Federation (Chonji forms)
- USTU - United States TKD Union (Tae Guek & Pal Gue forms)
- WTF - World TKD Federation (Tae Guek & Pal Gue forms)
- KTA - Korea TKD Association (Tae Guek & Pal Gue fo.Luts)

Nationally Recognized:

- USTF - United States TKD Federation (Chonji forms)
- USTA - United States TKD Alliance (Chonji forms)
- ATF - American TKD Federation (Chonji forms)
- USTA - United States TKD Association (Tae Geuk & Pal Gue forms)
- ATA - American TKD Association (Sang Anm forms)

☯ **Chapter 4**

Shopping for a Martial Arts School and Style

"Rank means nothing if the knowledge of these 'Masters' cannot help you achieve your goals."

Reasons Adults Study Martial Arts

At this point in the book, I've taken you through a journey covering the history of the martial arts, given you some insights into what it means to be successful in martial arts and how that can transcend every aspect of your life. I have provided a foundation for beginners in understanding the key elements of training of your body, mind, character and spirit. I have also provided an overview of the differences between some of the major styles to give you a better idea of your potential options depending upon where you live. There's only one thing missing – a place to do all of this and an instructor to take you on your journey to black belt and beyond.

So you're looking for a martial arts school or maybe you're looking for a school for your children. Either way there is a reason or motivation behind your desire to find a school. Understanding what you are looking for will make it easier to know when you have found it. As you begin your quest to find a suitable martial arts school that will meet your needs and expectations you will have many questions. There are many useful checklists in this chapter of what questions to ask instructors and yourself before you begin your personal journey into the martial arts.

The difficulty in shopping for a martial arts school is that as a non-martial artist, you are not qualified to evaluate the quality of the instruction. Assuming that your have no knowledge of martial arts, the information in this book will give you what you need to find a good school and to develop a better appreciation for what the martial arts are about.

What many potential students of martial arts focus on first are location, price and amenities. Yes, you want a school that is reasonably close to work or home and certainly you do not want to have to break the bank to afford it, but these are not the most important features. The quality of the instruction is paramount. You will be spending three or four days per week there if you are serious about improving and gaining what there is to gain, so ask a lot of questions; visit a lot of schools many times before making a choice. At the same time, keep in mind that sometimes your first martial arts school is like your first boyfriend or girlfriend. They may seem nice at first, but there's also a chance they just might not work and you should not let that negative experience keep you from trying again.

Shopping for a martial arts school is exciting and a little scary too. It's important to keep in mind that there are a wide variety of schools. A champion can be born in any environment. A school is simply a place to study and in the more traditional sense, it can even be outside where you don't even having four walls around you. Your school may be a garage or a corner of a gym or wherever. Don't think that the only schools worth attending are those that have the appearance of a modern club-like setting. While their appearance and accommodations may be tantalizing, the quality of instruction may not be of a high caliber.

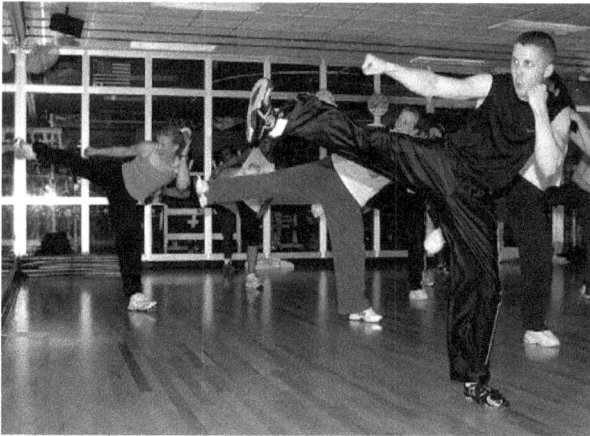

There are literally hundreds of martial arts styles from many countries. Pick up any copy of the Yellow Pages in any medium to large metropolitan area and you will likely see dozens of advertisements for martial arts schools. There are masters, grand masters, champions, world champions, senseis and sifus. There is Kung Fu, T'ai Chi, Judo, Tae Kwon Do, Shotokan, Aikido, Brazilian Jiu Jitsu, Karate Do, Kendo, Hapkido and many other "Do's" How can one sort them all out and begin to understand how to proceed?

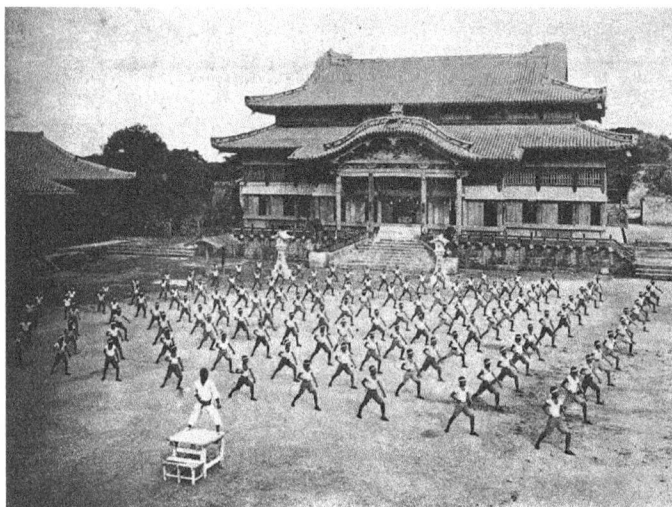

*A Traditional Martial Arts Class at Shuri Castle in Japan
1938 – no walls or cappuccino bars in this dojo!*

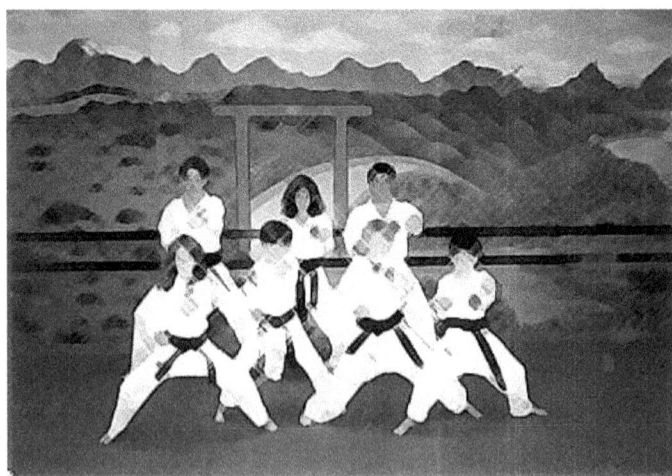

Black belts come in all sizes and ages!

Let's begin with understanding why you are looking for a martial arts school. What got you interested? What do you expect to get out of martial arts? There a number of reasons that people typically seek martial arts training for themselves or their children. In the box below are a few common reasons.

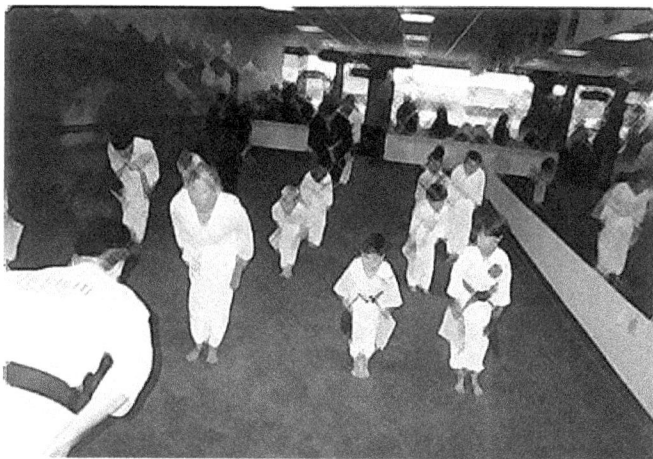

Respect and confidence are key qualities

Reasons Adults Study Martial Arts

1. I want to learn to defend myself.
2. I want a total body workout that includes cardio kickboxing instead of the typical workout at a local gym or health club.
3. I want to develop self-confidence, self-esteem, self-discipline.
4. I want to study martial arts traditions and styles as an art form.
5. I'm interested in Mixed Martial Arts (MMA).
6. I want to compete in martial arts tournaments.
7. I want to lose weight and get in shape.
8. I want to learn to become more focused (hey even adults need focus and structure!).
9. I want to become better at setting goals and achieving them.
10. I want to learn more about traditional martial arts values and ethics: humility, respect, honor, determination, perseverance, etc.

You may be motivated by one or more of these reasons or even something completely different. Regardless, there is a multitude of benefits to be gained from the study of martial arts. Take a few minutes and review the list above and identify which reasons are your main motivators. If your motivation is not on the list, write it down. Think these through and ask yourself, why the selected items are motivating you. I just want you to be sure of why you think you're interested in studying martial arts before you begin your search for an appropriate school.

Reasons Children Study Martial Arts

For our children, the common reasons for studying martial arts are similar. Parents may have motivations similar to those above and probably a number more as in the box below.

Reasons Children Study Martial Arts

1. I want my child to learn to defend himself/herself.
2. I want my child to become involved in a vigorous physical activity.
3. I want my child to develop self-confidence, self-esteem, self-discipline, respect.
4. I want my child to learn more about goal setting and personal achievement.
5. I want my child to learn traditional martial arts values and ethics: humility, respect, honor, determination, perseverance, and strength of character to stand up to peer-pressure or to confront bullying.
6. I want my child to learn to become better focused to help him or her out in school and to develop valuable life-skills.
7. My child needs more structure! (Don't we all!)

Again, review the list above and make sure you have a complete understanding of the reasons why you want your child studying martial arts and also what they're interest is. Often children will be motivated by television shows and movies they have seen where characters display impressive martial arts skills. If those are the visions they have swirling in their heads as they begin a martial arts program, so be it, as long as you, the parent, realize that the martial artists performing the stunts in the movies didn't learn those techniques overnight.

These two lists of reasons are pretty much carbon copies of virtually every advertisement you will ever see for any martial arts school. Somewhere in the promotional materials for any self-respecting school will be these key values, benefits and selling points. You the shopper must beware because while almost every school will claim to meet these needs, not all will really deliver the goods. Don't just assume that it's an automatic; insist.

This chapter will help you better understand what you should look for and ultimately what your study of the martial arts should include. If you study martial arts as they have been studied for centuries and learn the many qualities and skills that a true martial artist seeks to develop, you will achieve all of the objectives identified in the previous lists and have a rich and rewarding future in the martial arts.

At this point you have a list of reasons why you are interested in martial arts and what you hope to get out of it. Something to keep in mind however, is that martial arts and martial arts schools are not silver bullets. By that I mean that the instructors and curriculum and are not miracle cures for all that ails you or all that you hope to achieve. They can provide encouragement, structure and educate you to varying degrees on the basic values and qualities that will help you satisfy your needs. You will need to do much work to develop any skill, level or knowledge or personal qualities to reach the goals you have set for yourself or your child. Do not put all the burden or responsibility on the shoulders of your martial arts instructor. Before you start looking for a martial arts school there are a few more things you will need to consider in the following sections.

Martial Arts Benefits

In this section we'll take a brief look at benefits of martial arts study. I've already touched on many of the common benefits and outcomes that many people hope to gain from martial arts for themselves or their children. When you begin calling around or visiting martial arts schools I strongly recommend you make a list of your specific reasons. What is your "Why?" Whether you are shopping for yourself or your children, first make certain you know just what you are looking for. Review the list below and add any other reasons, benefits or desired outcomes you hope to gain from your adventure into the martial arts.

General Benefits of Martial Arts

1. Self-Confidence
2. Self-Defense
3. Self-Discipline
4. Physical Fitness
5. Improved focus and concentration
6. Respect for authority and others
7. Self-Respect
8. Achievement and Goal Accomplishment
9. Improved preparation and planning habits

The benefits listed above are just the highlights. Now you have given it some thought and hopefully have a better idea of what you are seeking. Let me assure you that once you find a suitable school, regardless of what reasons you have for studying the martial arts, I am certain you will find it invigorating and rewarding on many levels and you may even realize some benefits that you had never anticipated.

One side benefit of my study of martial arts is that when I first enrolled and earned my white belt, there was a very attractive blond in my white belt class who had signed up at the same time. She apparently had her eye on me while I was only focused on martial arts and developing the strength and stamina to continue on through the ranks with as much ease as she seemed to move along. Four years later we were married and four years after that we opened the United Karate Institute of Self Defense, Inc. in Alexandria, Virginia with three other instructors - not a bad side benefit. Certainly, I had not ever expected that signing up for martial arts would lead me to owning and managing a school and meeting my future wife. Signing up for martial arts was the best decision I ever made!

Qualities of a Martial Artist

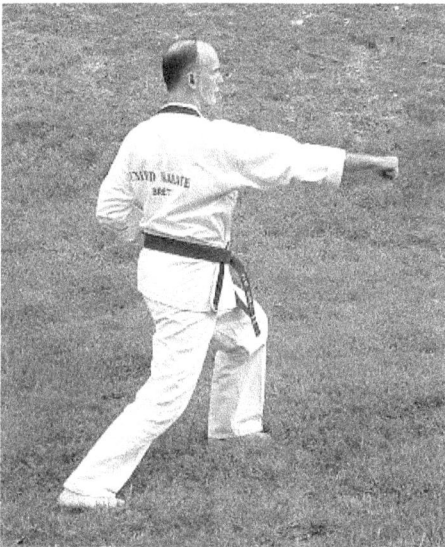

A well-rounded martial artist must learn about and focus on the following general topics of study:

Martial Arts Topics for Study and Development

- Martial Arts Origins and Traditions – *appreciation for the past*
- Skill and Training – *training the body*
- Strategy and Tactics – *training the mind*
- Spirit and Excellence – *training the soul and character*
- Success for Life – *foundations for the future!*

Within each of these general topic areas are dozens of sub-topics that make up the body of knowledge that a martial artist must learn and practice. It is a journey of a life-time and it can be life-changing. Martial arts really are about becoming what you were meant to be. Through martial arts training and the development of essential qualities, the potential for human development and achievement is unlimited!

Coincidentally the topics above are the chapters of my book The Way of the Martial Artist: Achieving Success in Martial Arts and in Life! I wrote that book because I wish I had a book like this when I began my martial arts studies. I would have progressed faster and farther and that is why I wrote it for my students.

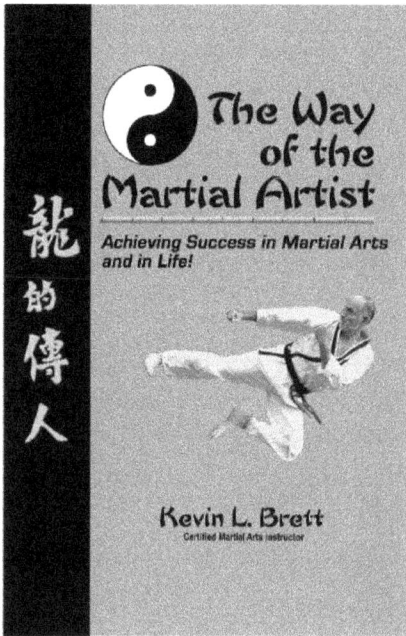

This book describes all of the essential qualities of a martial artist through each of the chapters in the box above and explains what these skills, techniques, strategies and concepts are to help you become a much better educated and enlightened martial artist. Feel free to go to my web site to read the actual Table of Contents, Foreword, Preface and Introduction. http://www.KevinBrettStudios.com

Martial Arts Instructors

As with school teachers, doctors, pilots, and any other profession, all martial arts instructors are not created equal. First of all, you have to remember martial arts are just that – an art form. Martial arts schools are not federally or state controlled. There is no consumer watchdog agency to ensure the quality or legitimacy of martial arts instruction. There are no national standards, criteria or requirements for martial arts. This is both a blessing and a curse. Essentially anyone can open a martial arts school after obtaining a business license.

Decent schools have instructors with a reasonable idea about what they are doing with their art and their teaching ability and at the same time also understand how to run the school as a business so they can pay the rent and keep the lights on. That being said, what does that tell you about their martial art, their ability to teach what you are looking for and the actual benefits that you will receive from studying with them; nothing much.

In the previous section there were a number of questions that I asked you answer about yourself and your reasons for wanting to study martial arts. In this section we'll address some of the questions you need to pose to the martial arts school instructors and owners

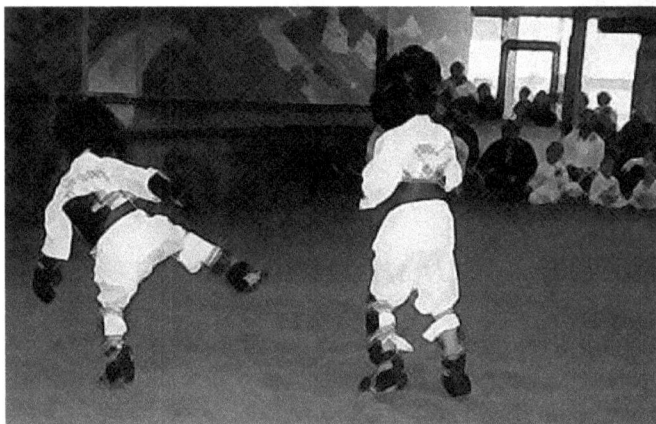

Mini-warriors learn control and self-discipline under pressure

First a few rules of thumb to consider: You will encounter many Masters and Grandmasters. Schools and their advertisements will tout their owner's amazing achievements in martial arts competition or in rank achievement. Many school owners will be high-ranking black belts such as 5th degree black belt up through 10th degree black belt. Every martial arts style has a slightly different scale of belts or colored sashes and ranks. Don't let this confuse, impress or intimidate you. Think of it as nothing more than some one who has gone through elementary school, then on to middle school, high school, college and possibly graduate school. ***Rank means nothing if the knowledge of these "Masters" cannot help you achieve your goals.***

All schools will claim to teach the standard fare: discipline, self-confidence, respect, etc. All schools will try to impress you with the qualifications and accomplishments of the owner or master, however, you will almost never be taught by that person, but by his or her junior instructors – often times you may be taught by an 18 year old who is a 1st degree black belt or sometimes even a brown belt. There is nothing inherently wrong with this as long as you do receive some instruction from higher ranking black belts as you increase in rank over time.

Some schools will tout the fact that they belong to some national or international association or federation related to their martial arts style. This is not a bad thing, but it is not a guarantee that you will receive quality instruction or that there will be good focus on self-defense or other key studies.

Most schools will try to fit you into what programs they have to offer. You want to try to pry more info out of them on how they will fit your needs and specifically how they will meet the claims that they make. Finally keep in mind that martial arts schools are not miracle factories. You will have to work and put a lot into it in order to get a lot out of it.

Questions for Martial Arts School
Instructors

1. How many instructors are on your staff?
2. What are their ages and qualifications or ranks?
3. How long have they been with you? (good schools will be good at retaining qualified and motivated instructor staff)
4. Are there any non-black belt level instructors teaching such as brown belts or red-belts? In other words, how much black belt instruction will I actually receive?
5. How do you train or qualify instructors? Are instructors simply those who have earned black belts or have they been through any type of instructor certification or training program beyond their basic black belt rank achievement?

Keep in mind that many schools may be staffed by one or two full-time instructors or school managers while the rest of the teaching staff is composed of part-time black belts who may not have been through any type of comprehensive instructor training or certification. This is where my comment earlier about all instructors not being created equal comes in. You must keep in mind that even if an instructor is certified by some means under someone that simply means they have had some type of training program that they have passed or through which they have earned some type of certificate. It does not mean they are skilled at teaching, gifted, motivated or even very competent. I must stress the importance here of visiting schools and watching several classes and how the different instructors interact with students at various belt ranks and skill levels. If a school will not allow you to observe their classes or answer questions about their instructors you probably want to pass on that organization.

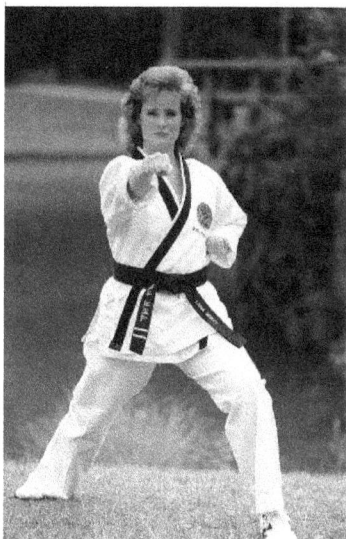

Any martial arts instruction should emphasize discipline and respect toward instructors and toward students as well as self-discipline. Instructors should be like an encouraging coach. There are times to be tough and times to be inspiring and motivating; watch for this. It is important to discuss with the instructors how they handle discipline. What methods do they use? Do they consider or handle input from parents, school teachers or other concerned parties. Discipline is important to reinforce respect and to provide boundaries for what is acceptable behavior, but it should not become an open door for verbal abuse or demeaning students. ***Discipline should be a learning experience and have a positive outcome that helps the student grow from the experience.***

While experience is important it is not the only thing that makes a good instructor. At United Karate we had one junior instructor who was eighteen and a first degree black belt. He was gifted with motivating children and keeping them under control, engaged and focused. Adults were also inspired by this young man. We put him through our 13 week instructor training and certification program complete with a 130 question practical exam. He was a better instructor than many higher ranking black belts I have come across.

In the box below is a list of some desirable traits you would hope to find in a good martial arts instructor. You will not necessarily find these qualities in *every* instructor, but during the course of your studies you will likely learn from multiple instructors and more senior martial artists and black belts. Make note of these qualities in the various instructors you encounter to determine which qualities you find most important and how the instructors seem to fit into these categories.

Instructor Qualities

1. Focused – doesn't get sidetracked from the lesson plan or the point that he or she is making.
2. Motivational – encourages everyone to dig deep and to want to work hard to improve.
3. Technically competent – must know the curriculum and be able to explain and break down techniques, kata/forms and all important strategies and concepts.
4. Knowledgeable – should have a reasonable grasp of the differences between major martial arts styles such as Chinese styles (Kung Fu, T'ai Chi), Korean Styles (Tae Kwon Do, Hapkido, Tang Soo Do, Mu Duk Kwon) Japanese Styles (Karate Do, Aiki Do, Kendo, Jiu Jitsu) Brazilian, Pilipino and so forth.
5. Disciplinary – able to maintain order, keep attention of the students, commands respect.
6. Technically skilled – able to demonstrate any and all techniques and concepts the way they should be performed.
7. Detail oriented – able to focus on small details of technique and performance.
8. Traditional – able to draw upon martial arts history, traditions and values and teach respect, humility, perseverance and many others essential qualities that all martial artists must develop.
9. Some instructors will expect students to condition themselves outside of class so that class time can be used to teach techniques while other instructors will use class time explicitly to help students physically train and condition. Both approaches have their pros and cons.

10. Instructors may or may not be in excellent physical shape, but they should be able to teach students how to properly execute techniques. Although it is generally a good sign when an instructor leads by example and is able to do exercises with the class at times. At other times it is important that the instructor is walking around observing as the class performs the exercises so that he or she can watch for proper technique and motivate students.

11. Instructors may or may not be in excellent physical shape, but they should be able to teach students how to properly execute techniques. Although it is generally a good sign when an instructor leads by example and is able to do exercises with the class at times. At other times it is important that the instructor is walking around observing as the class performs the exercises so that he or she can watch for proper

12. Good instructors explain the mechanics of movement and the physics of each technique. If they simply tell you to imitate them then you will never understand what you are doing and are likely to injure yourself.

13. Treats students with respect and encourages with positive motivation.

14. Love teaching martial arts and never tire of teaching.

15. Continue to improve their knowledge, skill and ability.

---

16. Instructors should ideally be able to demonstrate one or more lethal applications for any technique in a kata, unfortunately many were only taught some watered-down explanation for a technique or some symbolic interpretation. EVERY technique in a kata is for combat purposes. The ancient masters did not waste time or motion with fluff or superfluous techniques. To gain a better understanding of the concept of Bunkai (interpretation of kata), read my book or buy a copy of *"The Way of Kata"* by my friends Lawrence Kane and Kris Wilder. This book explains the REAL purpose of martial arts kata which 99% of commercial instructors are never taught.

Studying Options

Your martial arts studying options will be determined by the geography of where you live. Some areas will have a wider variety of options than others. Nonetheless, schools and training options can be generally categorized as shown below. Match these training options up to your reasons for studying martial arts from earlier in this chapter to get an idea of what you will be searching for in terms of a training experience.

Martial Arts Study Options
(types of schools)

1. Traditional Schools
2. Modern Schools with Sport Emphasis including mixed martial arts
3. Blended schools – with attention toward tradition, but also coverage of sport, competition, fitness training and self-defense applications
4. Self-Defense focused
5. Fitness-focused – cardio kickboxing
6. Weapons-focused schools/styles

Martial Arts Organizations and Associations

There are many martial arts clubs, associations and organizations in existence today. Many of these organizations function as the caretakers of their various styles and keep close watch over the teaching of these styles and the standards of performance and advancement.

It is important for students to understand the importance and the role that these organizations play in the martial arts world. To better understand the structure and role of these organizations it is useful to step back for a moment and consider the evolution of martial arts systems.

Finding the Right Martial Arts School for You

The martial systems that we study today are largely
derived from systems that were developed by
individuals. These individuals developed systems of self-
defense, gave them names, refined them and began to
teach them to others. Students of these instructors were
the proving ground for these martial systems and the
masters continued to refine, innovate and evolve their
systems and styles. As the systems developed into
maturity, various ranking schemes evolved with most of
them. Students were identified by their rank and
instructors could gauge their ability even without
personally knowing the student. As more curriculum
came into being, higher ranks were possible. Students
who stayed with a master for a long enough time could
rise in rank and skill as the master's own skill expanded
and the curriculum with it.

Various systems adopted sophisticated philosophical
and spiritual bases upon which they built their
techniques, strategies and customs. Like any family tree,
the martial arts family tree has many branches in many
countries. Each time a senior instructor would leave a
master, he would go to another location, teach what he
had learned and in many cases modify, innovate and
adapt his original system into a variant of what he had
mastered. In some cases, major innovations came into
existence by the hard work, analysis and creative insight
of masters who devised systems that were significantly
different from what they had originally learned.

Morehei Ueshiba, the founder of Aikido (meaning
"Harmony Way") built his system based on the
philosophy that he respected his opponent and
therefore wished no harm to his adversary. The original
techniques that he developed caused no permanent

harm to the adversary. There were no strikes or kicks that would inflict damage that would prevent an opponent from recovering after a time and coming back to continue an assault. I believe that philosophy, although honorable, is not a practical basis for a robust system of self-defense. Opponents will get up and return to the fight, at least until the defender has shown through enough attempts that he is impervious. Conversely, the general strategy in Kenpo Karate is to cause maximum damage in a complete flurry of devastating techniques. These styles of martial arts are on opposite ends of the force continuum.

Later variations of Aikido began to incorporate some number of simple kicks and strikes for use on a limited basis for persistent attackers. Later students of Ueshiba and his son developed these variations and they are now part of the martial family tree.

Tae Kwon Do and all of the other major and minor systems of martial arts have evolved, branched and morphed into a myriad of flavors all having some common elements. It is part of the martial tradition for a senior student to leave his master, go on his own, reflect and adapt and hopefully devise some useful innovations or potentially even introduce a radically new style or system. This keeps the arts dynamic, vibrant and growing.

In modern times, along with the development of new styles and systems comes the evolution of martial arts organizations and associations. These organizations charge membership and testing fees and provide some degree of quality assurance over their domain. Students derive a sense of legitimacy by receiving black belt certifications from them. Aside from revenue generation for the leaders of the organizations, certification and rank testing are usually promoted as providing acceptance for the students. If you obtain a black belt from organization "A", then you will be recognized anywhere that organization has a school or club. The problem with the recognition or certification is that many organizations refuse to recognize each other. These organizations typically require students to re-test on material that is very similar.

Often one organization may look upon black belts from another similar organization as being illegitimate. There are politics and egos involved and many organizations have come into being simply because the leadership of one organization had a falling out or fundamental differences so a divergence occurred and several new organizations then came into existence.

Another inconvenient feature of the organizations is that they periodically make subtle changes in the curriculum and the expected way in which the students are to perform the material. This is solely for requiring instructors to attend teaching seminars and to act as a control mechanism so that the organization maintains control over its affiliate schools. There are no practical, martial reasons for example, in changing how many Kihaps (yells) there are in a pattern, or on which moves they are to occur. This keeps instructors and students on their toes with useless and frivolous changes where time could be better spent focusing on the Bunkai (practical combat application), which most organizations do not teach or even know.

What are the advantages of these modern martial arts organizations? There is robust curriculum; however lacking it may be in specific focus on self-defense. These organizations are prevalent, instruction is usually consistent, and instructors do receive thorough training, which improves the student's experience. However, these martial organizations are highly politically charged often with much in-fighting. Self-defense and street survivability is often covered as more of an afterthought or an adjunct to the traditional curriculum, whereas if the focus were on the interpretation of the kata (Bunkai), then students would be learning what the movements of the patterns could do rather than learning to mimic a specific performance for purposes of passing a belt test. I have seen master-level classes where self-defense is not even discussed except in academic terms, not because there is any practical consideration of the need for it. The result, I believe, is students who are highly trained and tested in the tradition, etiquette, symbolic meanings and history of the kata and proper performance of techniques, but uneducated in the adaptation of these techniques and practical application for survival.

It is important for students to understand the importance and the role that these organizations play in the martial arts world. To understand better the structure and role of these organizations it is useful to step back for a moment and consider the evolution of martial arts systems.

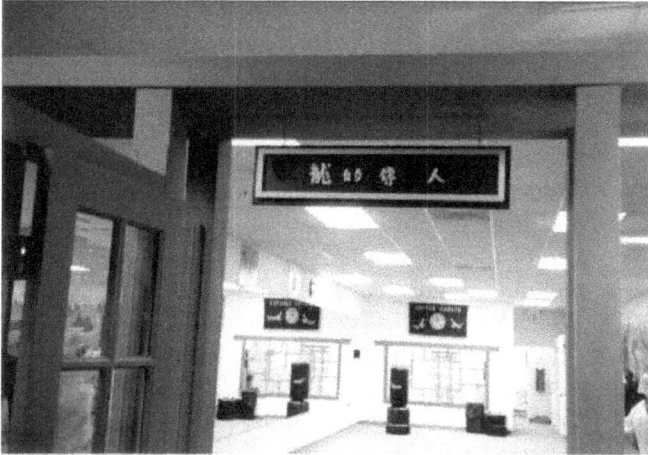

A view from the front entrance at United Karate. The weapons room is in the rear. The lettering is Chinese for "People of the Dragon" signifying wisdom, maturity and restraint.

Martial Arts Schools: Physical Layout

Martial arts schools vary in physical appearance, layout and accommodations greatly, but essentially a martial arts school is a big empty room. In fact, if you recall the photo of the Shuri Castle in Japan at the beginning of this chapter, you don't even necessarily need a room. Your dojo may be outside. Some schools are nicer, cleaner and equipped with more accommodations than others. But always remember that the quality of the instruction is the key factor. Location is probably second because you don't want to have to drive too far or you may be less motivated to stick with it. Some things that you may find or look for in a martial arts school are listed below.

Martial Arts School Accommodations

1. Bathrooms
2. Showers
3. Padded floors or large floor mats for throws and ground fighting
4. Large mirrors so that you can see how your techniques look
5. Weapons on racks (swords, bo-staffs)
6. Computerized billing and record keeping
7. A school web site
8. Customized school uniforms, gear and sports apparel
9. A pro shop
10. Books or videos for the school's curriculum
11. Weight equipment and other exercise equipment
12. Saunas and tanning beds
13. Handouts of the curriculum for each level
14. School vans for after school pickup (some schools have after school programs where they will help students with their homework
15. Adequate seating in the lobby – you will be spending time waiting for your children. Make sure you have a place to sit.

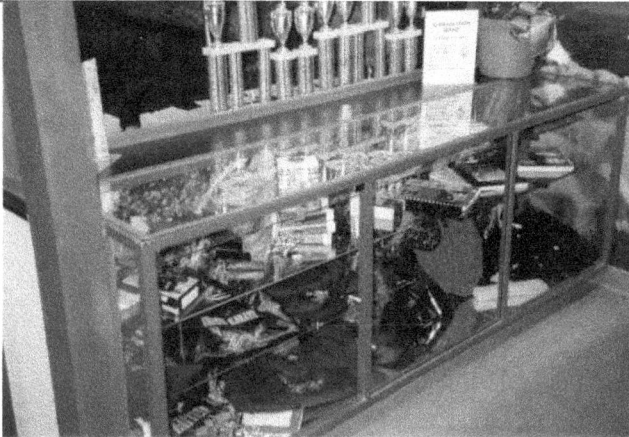

A display case with United Karate jackets, sparring gear, curriculum videos, student manuals and other goodies!

The essentials are simply a clean, safe room and the basic kicking and punching pads. It is not necessary to have a sauna, tanning beds or a juice bar or even showers. You will pay for these extras as part of your tuition. This leads to my next point: Where to find martial arts schools.

Where to Find Martial Arts Schools

1. Shopping malls
2. Strip malls
3. Universities
4. Asian book stores
5. Bulletin boards in martial arts supply stores
6. Churches
7. YMCA/YWCA
8. Community centers
9. Civic centers
10. Classified ads in newspapers
11. Yellow pages
12. Internet searches
13. Roadside signs
14. Word of mouth
15. Oriental restaurants
16. Local Military Bases
17. Local Police/Sheriff Departments

Martial Arts Programs

Before we discuss different types of programs that schools offer, let's talk about how schools might be run. Below are some key aspects of how a school might be structured to operate:

Individual classes for children and adults (occasionally, though, ages might be combined once or twice per week particularly on Saturday's when the schedule is shorter.)

Flexible schedule. For example if you are a yellow belt your schedule should offer a variety of times so that you can pick the

Sample Class Schedule	
Monday	5 PM
Tuesday	6 PM
Wednesday	7 PM
Thursday	8 PM
Friday	5 PM
Saturday	9 AM

days and times that fit your schedule. For any given belt rank, the schedule will vary something like the example above so that no matter what rank you are, you will have some variability in your schedule.

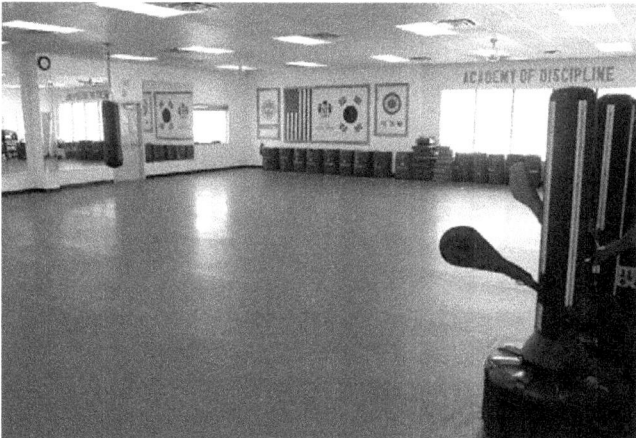

A typical Tae Kwon Do Dojang; flags, mirrors, pads, kicks pads along the far wall – the basics

School Program Features

1. Free intro class: Some schools have some type of introductory offer to allow you to have two or three classes or more so that you can try it out to see how you like the school. Often the intro offer will include a free uniform. However, the free uniforms are generally very light weight and inexpensive, so don't expect that uniform to last long. Once you have decided to get serious about your studies you should invest in a medium-weight uniform. As you become more advanced you may want a heavy weight uniform simply because they stand up better to the type of treatment that you will be giving them.

2. Some schools are also open on Sunday's, but that is much less common.

3. Open sparring or training sessions so that you can simply go and spar and workout. Ideally your school is large enough that maybe there is a second training room so that a class can be taking place in one room and other students can be practicing in another room.

4. Does your school actually have martial arts seminars by visiting martial artists? Many schools claim that is a benefit. A school that I belonged to for nine years claimed this and never offered a single seminar during the entire nine years! (and we inquired repeatedly).

5. Competition program: if you're into that

6. Separate self-defense classes that focus on realistic scenarios and training methods.

7. Separate weapons classes (generally for students who have been training for at least a year)

8. Demonstration team or a competition team to go to tournaments and demonstrations.

9. Programs for younger students ages 4-6 (Little Ninjas, Junior Dragons or something like that) Generally these are Karate-like classes where children will usually wear a uniform and maybe earn a white belt but not study and actual curriculum. These programs are generally intended as a feeder to the regular programs and allow younger children to begin to learn some basic martial arts concepts and activities.

10. Generally it should be allowable to come in and practice whenever the school is open as long as there is a practice room or space toward the back of the main room to practice as long as you are not disturbing the class.

Monthly: Pay as You Go

Monthly programs allow students to join and pay on a monthly basis without having to sign up for a one year or longer program. This provides flexibility so that if a student moves, changes schools or simply does not like the program a month or two into it; they are not stuck with a one-year membership. The disadvantage of this type of program is that over a longer period of time you will probably end up paying more than if you did sign up for a one year or longer program. There are always trade-offs.

If you sign up for some type of one year or longer program there will often be several payment methods:

School Payment Methods

1. **MONTHLY:** Make an initial deposit followed by monthly payments until the program fee has been paid off. (interest will almost always be included)
2. **QUARTERLY:** Make four equal payments four months in a row and the program is paid off. Obviously these four payments are larger than the 12 monthly payments mentioned above.
3. **PAY-IN-FULL:** One lump sum payment for the entire one year program. Usually some type of discount (10%) might be offered if you are paying in full.

Contracts: What to Expect

The first rule of contracts is **READ BEFORE YOU SIGN!** If you are not clear about what every single sentence in the contract means, get clarification so that you understand what you are getting into. Reading after you sign is too late!

Contracts will be written to provide the most flexibility and benefit for the school versus the student. That's simply how the business works. Read every line carefully and ask questions if you do not understand. Look for late fees, testing fees, belt fees, uniform costs, sparring equipment or any other requirements that might be part of the program. Find out if your program has a set time limit, such as one year, if it is possible to freeze the program. In other words, you may want to stop the clock for a few weeks if you know you will be out of town, or you become sick or injured or maybe just want a break without losing the time you have purchased. Often a program will say, for example, that you have one year or until you reach the rank of Blue Belt, whichever comes first. So if you are super dedicated like some students I have had, and earn your blue belt in six months, then your program is over and you have to sign up for the next level. On the other hand, if you spend a year training and you have not reached blue belt yet, your program is over. Either way this situation favors the school more than the student.

At United Karate, we did the opposite in order to favor the student. You could sign up for blue belt and you either had one year or you could continue to train beyond a year until you reached your blue belt. This positive policy actually resulted in more students staying with the program and ultimately accomplishing blue belt and continuing on to the black belt program. That is the goal of the school – retention of students. By favoring the students, you are actually favoring the school.

Schools will offer black belt programs and second degree black belt programs and masters or life programs. Each involves trade-offs which are based on whether you think you will stick with it or whether you are willing to make a long-term commitment. No one knows what the future holds. You may get transferred, become disabled, lose interest (ask if your program is transferable to another family member or someone else) or the school may go out of business. Not all martial arts schools are very financially stable. You will have to consider carefully which program suites your goals and tolerance for risk or uncertainty. (I sound like an

investment advisor here, but that's what you're doing –
making an investment).

Location, Location, Location

You've heard that saying before. What I mean by this is
that there are many locations or places to find a martial
arts school. You may find a school at the YMCA, or
within a sports club or a county recreation center. Your
school may be located within a local strip mall shopping
center or inside of a larger enclosed mall. It really does
not matter where it is located as long as it is in a safe
neighborhood and is a clean and reasonably spacious
facility. I've already said this but it bears repeating, that
you need to go watch several classes on several different
occasions to see how they are run and how different
instructors interact with students and how they control
and motivate their classes.

Costs

Martial arts are an art form, but they are also a business.
Someone has to pay to keep the lights on. That being
said, there are a variety of ways that schools generate
revenue and keep the cash flowing in. This is not a bad
thing, but you need to be aware of the various costs that
you will likely incur on your journey.

Martial Arts Costs and Fees

1. Uniform (good idea to have two)
2. Sparring gear. Padded head gear, mouth guard, hand, feet, shins and chest guard.
3. Testing fee (each belt level may require a test fee before you can graduate to the next belt level. This is in addition to your regular membership or program fee.
4. Seminar fees (unless they are included in the program contract)
5. Weapons (advanced students often purchase practice weapons such as foam nunchukas, or wood or bamboo swords or rubber knife or wooden gun for self-defense practice.
6. Tournament or competition fees (not generally part of your school)
7. If your school is part of a national or international affiliation such as the U.S. Tae Kwon Do Federation, or the World Tae Kwon Do Federation, then there may be separate annual membership fees or testing fees. Inquire about these fees or see if these are included in the membership at your school.
8. After school fees if you participate in one of these programs at the school.

The Art of Shopping!

Now you are ready to begin your search. In the next few boxes below are a few key considerations when you visit a school:

Tips for Visiting a School

1. Be respectful and polite. Respect is the first lesson in martial arts. Without it learning cannot take place.
2. Shake hands if an instructor offers to shake hands
3. If someone bows to you, bow back out of respect.
4. Call the school to find out if visitors are allowed to come and watch.
5. If there are high-pressure sales tactics, you don't want to be there.
6. Observe the classes quietly to show respect and not to distract the students or the instructors.
7. Do not try to impress anyone with what you have learned about martial arts in your reading. Focus on learning what you can.
8. Try to avoid discussing other schools you have visited; just focus on learning about the one you're in at the moment.
9. Classes will vary greatly from day to day and from instructor to instructor. Go observe many classes at the schools that seem to be on your short list. Every instructor has a bad day once in a while so watch enough classes to get a good idea. You may show up on a day when they are teaching weapons or self-defense only. The more classes you watch the better sampling you have to make your judgment.
10. Find out when enrollment is possible. Commercial schools will generally start any time. University programs or community centers will only start every six weeks or every semester. Check ahead of time.

I spoke wrote earlier about various styles of martial arts. There are also various ways of training in a given martial art. Below is a list of potential training styles that you should ask about to determine if the school teaches in a manner that is within your comfort zone. On the other hand, martial arts is about leaving your comfort zone and stretching your abilities to achieve new heights! But here's the list anyway:

Training and Sparring Styles

1. Traditional – generally focusing on forms, kata, hyungs, poomse
2. Mixed Martial Arts – combination of various styles including boxing, grappling, wrestling and other striking arts – more or less the opposite of traditional
3. Sport Karate – involves light contact point sparring
4. Olympic-style – involves semi-contact
5. Full-contact – usually requires a tough personality and body
6. Self-Defense – focusing on realistic, practical street techniques without much study of an established martial art system

---

School Atmosphere

1. Are students and instructors respectful toward each other?
2. Do the instructors appear to enjoy teaching or do they look like they can't wait for class to end?
3. Do students appear to be enjoying themselves?
4. Is the class fun but serious or is there too much joking around and silliness? It's ok to have some levity, but martial arts are a serious topic.
5. Do instructors pay attention to details; teaching concepts as well as the mechanics of a technique?

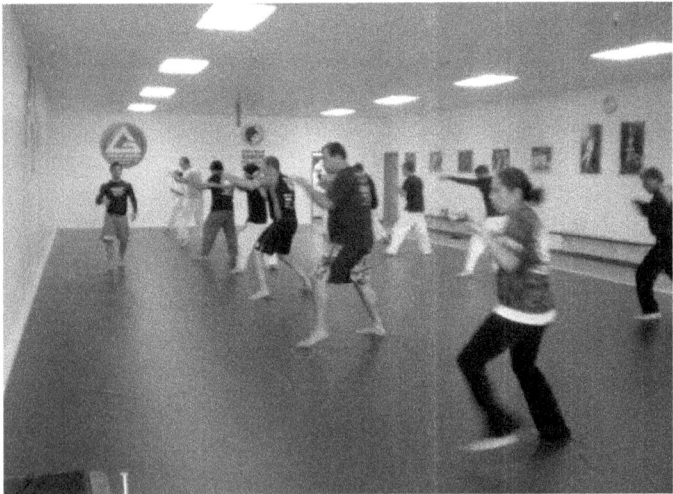

A mixed martial arts class working out in their dojo

The Best Style of Martial Art

I am always amused when I hear someone ask what is the best style of martial art. There is no best martial art. They are all intended to focus on self-defense. The key is whether or not your training really focused on the reality of combat and self-defense in realistic scenarios and settings or just on memorization of forms/kata/hyungs/poomse and training for competition and sport karate.

If you do a Google search on "Bunkai" you will find that it is a Japanese term meaning interpretation of kata or forms. What 99% of martial arts schools teach in their kata is what really well versed martial artists refer to as the "B" knowledge. These are watered-down or made up explanations of how to use various moves from the kata. The kata or forms are simply the vocabulary of the given style. Like any language, you learn the vocabulary and basic structure and then you learn to write your own thoughts. In other words, on the street you would never jump in and begin to execute a green belt form, but you would use some of the moves from it (if you have studied the "A" knowledge through bunkai") to defend yourself.

A simple movement like a front-stance with a down-block is typically taught as blocking a roundhouse kick from your opponent. Try this for real and you will end up with a broken forearm. Which is stronger, your forearm or your opponent's shin? In reality a movement like that is intended to defend against someone who has grabbed your forearm. Step BACKWARDS, not forwards as you typically do in a kata, wrap around with the arm being grabbed and re-grab your opponent's forearm, while stepping back into your front stance, then down block against the back of their elbow as you drop your weight down suddenly into your front stance. The end result is your opponent has a broken or hyper extended elbow and will not be giving you any trouble for quite some time.

I realize this is difficult to visualize in written form, but the point is that every movement in a Tae Kwon Do form or any other form of any other style actually has three or four or many practical and often lethal applications if you spend enough time learning from someone who knows the kata. So take the movements you already know and study their practical application before going into another style of martial art and repeating the same behavior.

As far as other styles however, there are some that do come across a little more intuitive in the self-defense arena: Hapkido, Ed Parker Style Kenpo Karate, Jiu Jitsu, Krav Maga, to name a few. But again, any style can be effective if you are taught effectively. It depends up on how much knowledge you have about how to use the techniques you have learned.

When it comes to children, there are children who study Judo, Kendo (swordsmanship), various of the Chinese styles such as Wu Shu, Kung Fu and so forth. Clearly the most prevalent in the United States is Tae Kwon Do or one of the similar Japanese or Okinawan styles of Karate or Isshin Ryu (Ryu means school). What is good about these styles is that children can develop proficiency relatively easily and if they are taught with a self-defense emphasis as they get into their middle-school years, then they can apply these skills in a real situation if needed.

You must learn about many topics which I cover in my book *"The Way of the Martial Artist"* to be fully versed and prepared for self-defense whether it is in a parking lot or in Iraq. You must understand principles of camouflage, concealment and evasion. You must learn how to use your environment and terrain to your advantage. You must learn about weapons of opportunity; how to use what is at your disposal and within arm's reach to defend your self – and actually practice this vs. just reading about it. There are tactics and strategies and training methods that I discuss which will allow you to take what you have learned in the martial arts school and help you make it work in combat. That is the purpose of it all.

More important than any specific techniques are the proper knowledge, mindset and spirit. You must understand the real meanings of terms like timing and speed and how to isolate the difference between them in drills so that you can improve these qualities. You must develop a "survivor" mindset that also involves understanding of how you would truly react and what your triggers would be in a self defense situation. Where is your "line of conviction"? How far can someone push you before you react and then where will you enter into the force continuum. When we were operating our martial arts school United Karate Institute of Self Defense, Inc. we had a slogan that said it all:

"If you can't defend yourself . . . nothing else matters."

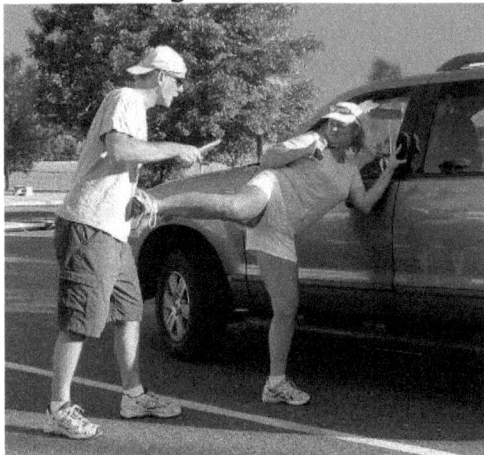

Shopping Around

I have said many things about what to look for and what to expect from a martial arts school and your journey in the martial arts. There is no single school or instructor that will be perfect in every aspect. Do not think that because some aspects of a school, instructor or program may not meet every criteria perfectly that it is not a good school. Many schools will stack up about the same on any list of criteria or questions.

My goal is writing this book is the help you become familiar with what can be expected and what should be expected of you or your child so that you are a better educated student going into your martial arts experience. As you review this beginner's guide and visit schools and read about martial arts styles, you will become better at being able to differentiate between different schools and eventually make a good choice. Do not rush! Take your time so that you will find a school that will really be right for you. Re-read this book to review key points and then begin your search, but at some point, you must commit if you are ever going to begin your personal journey.

My experience has been that, generally speaking, many commercial schools are fairly similar in what they offer, what they cost and the quality of instruction that you receive. Some are considerably better in various areas and that is why you need to take your time and discover these differences.

You will need to do a lot of study on your own as you should in any academic or artistic endeavor. Read books, buy videos, surf the internet and check out martial arts magazines. There is much to learn and you will not find all of it at your school, but it should be your home base where you put into practice what you have learned. Do no rely on a single instructor to be your sole source of martial arts knowledge or training. There is too much out there to learn, experience and enjoy so don't limit yourself.

Train hard and with good spirit. You are the next generation of martial arts!

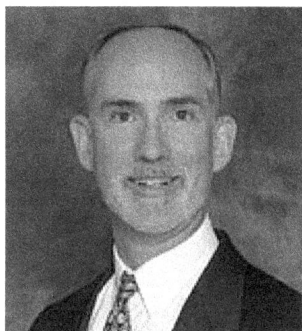

About the Author

Kevin Brett is a certified martial arts instructor with twenty years of martial arts training and teaching experience. He and wife Lana Kaye Brett were two of the five co-founders of the United Karate Institute of Self-Defense, Incorporated in Alexandria, Virginia. He has taught martial arts and street self-defense to local law enforcement, military and federal officers focusing on realistic and practical application of martial arts techniques. He has studied Tae Kwon Do, Jiu Jitsu, Kendo, Kenjutsu, Kenpo Karate, Shotokan, Aiki Do and many other styles to add to his diverse experience base.

He is the President/CEO of Kevin Brett Studios, Inc., and the author of *The Way of the Martial Artist: Achieving Success in Martial Arts and in Life!* and *"Journey to Black Belt: Begin the Journey to Transform Your Life!"* Information and samples from these comprehensive martial artist's books can be viewed at www.KevinBrettStudios.com

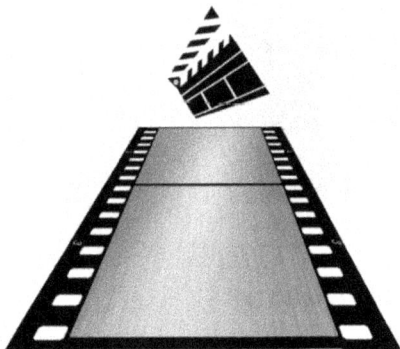

Entertainment | Education | Family

www.KevinBrettStudios.com

Appendix A: Listing of Internet Martial Arts School Directories

Below are the top ten martial arts school directories on the internet. Certainly a quick Google search can also help you find more schools in your area as well. Don't forget to check other possible avenues of locating a school as mentioned in the last chapter in the list titled "Where to Find Martial Arts Schools"

Martial Arts School Directories
http://www.martialdirect.com/Category/Directory-Listings/
http://www.dojos.com/directory.htm
http://www.dojolocator.com/
http://www.masites.com/schools.cfm
http://www.martialinfo.com/search.asp
http://www.martialartslistings.com/
http://www.usadojo.com/kata/schools.asp
http://www.martialartschoolsdirectory.com/
http://www.martialedge.net/martial-arts-school-directory/
http://www.martialschools.com/

www.ingramcontent.com/pod-product-compliance
Lightning Source LLC
Chambersburg PA
CBHW070534030426
42337CB00016B/2196